NATURAL HAIR AND SKINCARE REMEDIES

(VOLUME I: HAIR REMEDIES)

By
Brittany M Robinson

Natural Hair And Skin Care Remedies

(Volume I: Hair Remedies)

Copyright © 2022 by Brittany M Robinson

Published By: Brittany M Robinson

Printed in the United States of America

ISBN: 979-8-9862607-1-6(Hardcover)

979-8-9862607-4-7(Paperback)

For information Contact:

Mrs. Robinson Natural Solutions at

Http://mrsrobinsonnaturalsolutions.com

All natural products to make your hair healthier and grow faster. Keep your hair healthy by using natural products. Butter and oil are healthy for your hair and body.

A little about me – I'm a happily married, Mother of 4. I got the inspiration for my book from my children.

Skin and body rash sometime an inflammation of the skin. You might see a change in color of the skin or texture. Rashes could irritation the skin or allergic reaction. Allergies could be due to food, plants, chemicals, animals, insects, and environmental. Skin rash could affect the entire body or area of the body. Eruptions on the skin of the back are called Back Rash. Even though All rashes are not contagious, some could be.

One day, I noticed my son, JerMichael, had got some rashes; I used different types of products for a few months, but it didn't help. The rashes on his body were very serious; and the doctor said that we should not apply any products without knowing what in the products. It can put your children in great danger of skin-related issues. After that, I studied it, and I believe there are a lot of people out there who are facing the same issue.

After spending thousands of dollars on different products, this book includes all the tips and steps I tried in getting rid of my son's rashes. If you purchase this book, you can save thousands of dollars or hundreds of hours, as I've wasted mine to help you. I started making my own natural body wash, oils, butter, and, body pain oils. The rash you are experiencing may have a different root than my son's. However, I believe this book can help you.

Table of Contents

When using the hair products, you can substitute any oils, butter, and wax.

In the back of the book, it is going to have different butter and oils that you can substitute to know if your hair is Low or High Porosity. Put a strand of clean hair in a glass of water, and let it sink to the bottom of your hair with high porosity. If your hair strand floats to top and take a while to sink, it is low porosity.

If your strand hair midway in glass, it is normal porosity.

Things you will need before you start making your homemade products.

- Glass Blender or stick blender
- Whisk
- Food processor
- Bowls
- Pots
- Funnel
- Cutting board
- Wooden spoon
- Grinder
- Containers
- Bottles
- Measurement cups

If you have an itching scalp, this will give you relief. Cornstarch and baking soda help with itching scalp, if your hair is itching or allergic, try this remedy.

1. Just mix a quarter of Cornstarch and 1 teaspoon baking soda, put it in a store-able container.
2. Sprinkle small amount in your hair and scalp. This also helps to remove grease hair.
3. Leave it for 30 minutes, then rinse out your hair.

Itchy Scalp Spray

Apple vinegar cleanses your scalp and help your hair growth and balance your Hp.

1. 2tsp Apple vinegar.
2. Put it in the spray bottle, add distilled water in the bottle spray, then spray it on your scalp.
3. Leave it for 15-20 minutes, then wash it out.

Basic Hair Butter

Ingredients:

- 6 tsp. of cocoa butter or mango butter
- 3 tsp. of jojoba oil
- 3 tsp. of honey
- 1 tsp Ayurveda oil (hair Growth oil)
- 5 drop tea tree essential oil

Directions:

1. Use a double-boiler to melt cocoa butter and jojoba oil.
2. After the cocoa butter and the jojoba oil are completely melted, add honey to the mixture.
3. Let the mixture cool until it hardened.
4. Before it gets hardened, whip it (until it looks like whipped cream texture) about 4-5 minutes.
5. Then add 5 drops of essential oil (optional)
6. Put it in the container.

Cupuacu Hair Butter Cream

Ingredients:

- ½ cup cupuacu butter
- ¼ cup jojoba oil
  ¼ cup Mango butter
- 2 tbsp almond oil
  2 tbsp of castor oil
- 20 lemongrass essential oil
- 20 rosemary essential oil

Directions:

1. Melt butter in a double boil.
2. Put it in the refrigerator until solid, then add oils, and use your hand mixer (thick butter, it will take 5 minutes or more) It will look creamy.
3. Add essential oils and mix it until smooth.
4. Pour it into a jar.

Murumuru and Cocoa Hair Butter

Ingredients:

- 6 tsp. of murumuru butter
- 3tsp. Cocoa butter
- 3 tsp. of argan oil
- 3 tsp. of rose hip oil
- 1 tsp pomegranate oil
- 5 drops peppermint essential oil
- 5 drops rosemary essential oil

Directions:

1. Use a double-boiler to melt murumuru, cocoa butter, and oils.
2. After the murumuru, cocoa butter and the oils are completely melted, let the mixture cool until hardened.
3. Before it gets hardened, whip it (until it looks like whipped cream texture) for about 4-5 minutes.
4. Then add 5 drops of essential oil (optional).
5. Put it in a container.

Shea Butter and honey Hair cream

Ingredients:

- 6 tsp. of Shea butter
- 3 tsp. of sunflower
- 3 tsp. of honey
- 1 tsp. Argan oil
- 5 drop rosemary essential oil

Directions:

1. Use a double-boiler to melt shea butter and argan oil.
2. After the shea butter and the argan oil are completely melted, add honey to the mixture.
3. Let the mixture cool until it hardens.
4. Before it gets hardened, whip it (until it looks like whipped cream texture) for about 4-5 minutes.
5. Then add 5 drops of essential oil.
6. Put it in a container.

kokum Hair Butter

Ingredients:

- 6 tsp. of kokum butter
- 3 tsp. of argan oil

- 3 tsp. of almond oil
- 1 tsp Babassu oil
- 5 drops lemongrass essential oil
- 5 drops lavender essential oil

Directions:

1. Use a double-boiler to melt kokum butter and oils.
2. After the kokum butter and the oils are completely melted, let the mixture cool until it hardened.
3. Before it gets hardened, whip it (until it looks like whipped cream texture) for about 4-5 minutes.
4. Then add 5 drops of essential oil (optional).
5. Put it in a container.

Tamanu and Mango hair butter

Ingredients:

- 6 tsp. of Tamanu butter
- 6tsp mango butter
- 3 tsp. of argan oil
- 3 tsp. of vitamin E oil
- 1 tsp grapeseed oil
- 5 drops sweet orange essential oil
- 5 drops vanilla essential oil
- 5 drops cinnamon essential oil

Directions:

1. Use a double-boiler to melt tamanu, mango butter and oils.
2. After the tamanu, mango butter and the oils are completely melted, let the mixture cool until it hardened.
3. Before it gets hardened, whip it (until it looks like whipped cream texture) for about 4-5 minutes.
4. Then add 5 drops of essential oil (optional).
5. Put it in a container.

Avocado hair Butter

Ingredients:

- 6 tsp. of Avocado butter
- 6tsp. Cocoa butter
- 3 tsp. of argan oil
- 3 tsp. of sunflower oil
- 1 tsp bhringraj powder
- 1tsp fenugreek powder
- 1tsp amla powder
- 5 drops rosemary essential oil

Directions:

1. Use a double-boiler to melt avocado, cocoa butter and oils.
2. After the avocado, cocoa butter and the oils are completely melted, add the bhringraj, fenugreek and amla.
3. Let the mixture cool until it hardened.
4. Before it gets hardened, whip it (until it looks like whipped cream texture) for about 4-5 minutes.
5. Then add 5 drops of essential oil.
6. Put it in a container.

Cocoa Hair Butter

Ingredients:

- 6tsp. Cocoa butter
- 6tsp Mango butter
- 3 tsp. of argan oil
- 3 tsp. of safflower oil
- 1tsp vitamin E oil
- 5 drops lavender essential oil

Directions:

1. Use a double-boiler to melt Mango, cocoa butter and oils.
2. After the Mango, cocoa butter and the oils are completely melted, add the safflower and 1tsp vitamin E.
3. Let the mixture cool until it hardened.
4. Before it gets hardened, whip it (until it looks like whipped cream texture) about 4-5 minutes.
5. Then add 5 drops of essential oil.
6. Put it in a container.

Moringa and fenugreek Cocoa Hair Butter

Ingredients:

- 6 tsp. Of cocoa butter
- 3 tsp. of argan oil
- 3 tsp. of sunflower oil
- 1 tsp moringa powder
- 1tsp fenugreek powder
- 5 drop sweet orange essential oil

Directions:

1. Use a double-boiler to melt cocoa butter and oils.
2. After the avocado, cocoa butter and the oils are completely melted, add moringa and fenugreek.
3. Let the mixture cool until it hardened.
4. Before it gets hardened, whip it (until it looks like whipped cream texture) for about 4-5 minutes.
5. Then add 5 drops of essential oil.
6. Put it in a container.

Aloe vera and rose water hair gel

Ingredients:

- 4 oz distill water
- 2 oz rose water
- 2 tsp. Glycerin
- 3 tsp. of aloe vera powder
- 1 tsp guar gum
- 1 tsp clear Xanthan gum (cosmetic grade)
- 1 tsp Xanthan gum
- 2g Leucidal liquid SF

Directions:

1. Put your clear xanthan gum and glycerin in a bowl and stir it with a spoon. Put it aside for 35minutes.

2. Then pour the distilled water and rose water in the aloe vera powder then add Leucidal liquid and stir it.

3. Get the xanthan gum and glycerin and gradually add the water.

4. Let it sit for 1 hour, it should look like a gel.

5. Put it a container.

6. Apply it in your hair.

Making Candle Hair and Skin Butter

Ingredients:

- 1cup Cocoa Butter
- ½ cup Mango Butter
- 2tsp emulsify wax or beeswax
- 1tsp jojoba oil or castor oil
- 1tsp olive oil
- 1tsp vitamin E
- 5 drops rosemary essential oil(option)
- 10 drops lavender essential oil (option)
- 1tsp henna (optional). Don't use it on your skin, it is only for hair growth

Directions:

1. Use a double boiler to mix Butter and wax until it melts (low heat). It will take a long time for the wax to melt, give it time.
2. Add 1tsp jojoba oil, Henna is optional, then add 5 drops rosemary oil, add 10 drops lavender oil, then put your wicks inside your jar then pour your mixture until it hardens.

3. Now you can burn your wicks and let the oil melt and apply in your hair. Don't apply when it is too hot.

Avocado & Macadamia Candle Hair Butter

Ingredients:

- 1 cup Avocado Butter
- 1 cup Macadamia
- 2tsp Yellow beeswax
- 1tsp vitamin E
- 1tsp Almond oil
- 1tsp honey
- 5drops cedarwood oil(optional)
- 1tsp Moringa Powder (optional)

Directions:

1. Use a double boiler to make a mixture of butter and wax. It will take longer to melt.
2. Add the almond oil, moringa, essential oil, then place your wick in the jar then pour your mixture and let it sit overnight.
3. Now you can burn it and use the butter for your hair.

Kokum Candle hair Butter

Ingredients:

- 1 cup kokum Butter
- 2tsp Yellow beeswax
- 1tsp vitamin E
- 1tsp sunflower oil
- 1tsp honey
- 5 drops lavender essential oil
- 5 drop vanilla essential oil

Directions:

1. Use a double boiler to make a mixture of butter and wax. It will take longer to melt.
2. Add the sunflower oil, honey, vitamin E, essential oil, then place your wick in the jar then pour your mixture and let it sit overnight.
3. Now you can burn it and use the butter for your hair.

Avocado and cocoa Candle hair butter

Ingredients:

- 1 cup Avocado Butter
- 1 cup cocoa butter
- 2tsp Yellow beeswax
- 1tsp vitamin E
- 1tsp Argan
- 1tsp sunflower
- 5drops lemongrass essential oil
- 5drop sweet orange essential oil

Directions:

1. Use a double boiler to make a mixture of butter and wax. It will take longer to melt.
2. Add the argan, sunflower and essential oil, then place your wick in the jar then pour your mixture and let it sit overnight.
3. Now you can burn it and use the butter for your hair.

Peppermint Tucuman Candle Hair Butter

Ingredients:

- 1 cup Tucuman Butter
- 2tsp Yellow beeswax
- 1tsp vitamin E
- 1tsp sunflower oil
- 1tsp honey
- 10 drops peppermint essential oil

Directions:

1. Use a double-boiler to make a mixture of butter and wax. It will take longer to melt.
2. Add the vitamin E, honey and essential oil, then place your wick in the jar and pour your mixture and let it sit overnight.
3. Now you can burn it and use the butter for your hair.

Shea Butter hair Candle

Ingredients:

- 1 cup Shea Butter
- 1 tsp jojoba oil
- 2tsp Yellow beeswax
- 1tsp vitamin E
- 1tsp rose hip oil
- 1tsp honey
- 5 drops rose jasmine essential oil
- 5 drops bergamot essential oil

Directions:

1. Use a double-boiler to make a mixture of butter and wax. It will take longer to melt.
2. Add the jojoba, vitamin E, honey, rose hip, essential oil, then place your wick in the jar then pour your mixture and let it sit overnight.
3. Now you can burn it and use the butter for your hair.

Gingerbread Candle hair Butter

Ingredients:

- 1 cup Kokum Butter
- 1 cup Avocado butter
- 2tsp Yellow beeswax
- 1tsp vitamin E
- 1tsp argan oil
- 1tsp sunflower oil
- 6 drops vanilla essential oil (optional)
- 6 drops clove essential oil
- 10 drops ginger essential oil or 1 tsp ground ginger
- 6 drops of cinnamon essential oil or 1tsp ground cinnamon

Directions:

1. Use a double-boiler to make a mixture of butter and wax. It will take longer to melt.
2. Add the sunflower, argan, and essential oils.
3. Then place your wick in the jar and pour your mixture and let it sit overnight.
4. Now you can burn it and use the butter for your hair.

Sugar Cookie Candle

Ingredients:

- 1 cup cocoa Butter
- ½ cup granulated sugar
- 2tsp Yellow beeswax
- 1tsp vitamin E
- 1tsp Argan oil
- 1tsp sunflowers oil
- 1tsp sprinkles
- 20 drops very vanilla candle scent
- 40 drops vanilla fragrance oil

Directions:

1. Use a double-boiler to make a mixture of butter and wax. It will take longer to melt.
2. Add the Sugar, sunflowers, sprinkles essential oil, then place your wick in the jar then pour your mixture and let it sit overnight.
3. Now you can burn it and use the butter for your hair.

Palm & Mango Candle Hair Butter

Ingredients:

- 1 cup Mango Butter
- 1 cup Palm butter
- 2tsp Yellow beeswax
- 1tsp sunflower oil
- 1tsp argan oil
- 1tsp honey
- 1 tsp Morocco
- 5 drops ginger essential oil
- 5 drops vanilla essential oil
- 5 drops cinnamon essential oil

Directions:

1. Use a double-boiler to make a mixture of butter and wax. It will take longer to melt.
2. Add the sunflower, argan, honey, Morocco essential oil, then place your wick in the jar then pour your mixture and let it sit overnight.
3. Now you can burn it and use the butter for your hair.

Vanilla Pumpkin Pie Candle

Ingredients:

- 1 cup Mango Butter
- 1 cup Cocoa butter
- 2tsp Yellow beeswax
- 1tsp sunflower oil
- 1tsp argan oil
- 1tsp Olive squalene
- 2 tsp pumpkin spice
- 5 drops ginger essential oil
- 5 drops nutmeg essential oil
- 5 drops cinnamon essential oil

Directions:

1. Use a double-boiler to make a mixture of butter and wax. It will take longer to melt.
2. Add the sunflower, argan, Pumpkin spice and essential oil, then place your wick in the jar then pour your mixture and let it sit overnight.
3. Now you can burn it and use the butter for your hair.

Pumpkin Spice Hair Candle

Ingredients:

- 1 cup Shea Butter
- 2tsp Yellow beeswax
- 1tsp sunflower oil
- 1tsp argan oil
- 5 drops ginger essential oil
- 5 drops vanilla essential oil
- 5 drops cinnamon essential oil
- 5drop nutmeg oil
- 5 drop orange oil

Directions:

1. Use a double boiler to make a mixture of butter and wax. It will take longer to melt.
2. Add the sunflower, argan, essential oil, then place your wick in the jar then pour your mixture and let it sit overnight.
3. Now you can burn it and use the butter for your hair.

Moisturizing Sealing Tucuman Butter Recipe for hair

Ingredients:

- 4 oz Tucuman butter
- 2 teaspoons Argan oil
- 2 teaspoons jojoba oil
- 2 teaspoon Marula oil
- 2 teaspoon Grapeseed oil
- 10 drop essential patchouli oil (optional)

Directions:

1. Melt butter in a double boiler.
2. Put it in the refrigerator until it becomes solid then, add oils, and use your hand mixer.
3. Add essential oils and mix them until smooth.
4. Pour it into a jar. Your butter is ready, and it's time to style your hair.

Goats Milk Soap condition bars

Ingredients:

- 140g Goats Milk Soap Base Melt
- 2 tablespoon Cocoa Butter
- 2 tablespoon grade seed Oil
- 1 tablespoon Sweet Almond Oil
- 1/2tsp Vitamin E Oil
- Add 5 to 10 drops Vanilla Essential Oil (optional)
- Soap molds

Directions:

1. Melt goat Milk base soap in the crockpot (or double boiler), then add cocoa butter.
2. When the Goat Base and cocoa butter completely melt, add oils.
3. Add vanilla and pour the mixture in soap molds.
4. Once the soap bars are hardened, you can pop them out.

Argan soap condition bars

Ingredients:

- 140g Argan Soap Base Melt
- 2 tablespoon Cocoa Butter
- 2 tablespoon sunflower oil
- 1/2tsp Vitamin E Oil
- Add 10 drops Chamomile oil
- 10 lavender essential oil
- Soap molds

Directions:

1. Melt goat Argan soap in the crockpot (or double boiler), then add cocoa butter.
2. When the Argan Base and cocoa butter completely melt, add oils.
3. Add essential oil and pour the mixture in soap molds.
4. Once the soap bars are hardened, you can pop them out.

Winter shampoo bar

Ingredients:

- 1 cup White soap base
- 1 tsp Vitamins E
- 1 tsp jojoba oil
- 10 drops sandalwood essential oil
- 10 drops geranium essential oil
- 6 drops bergamot

Directions:

1. Put the crockpot, add soap base, and oil; stir it until it melts.
2. Add oils and mix it until it melts.
3. Add essential oil, keep stirring it.
4. Pour it in the mold and allow it to harden and pop them out.

Aloe Vera Soap condition bars

Ingredients:

- 140g Aloe vera glycerin
- 2 tablespoon argan oil
- 1 tablespoon jojoba oil
- 1/2tsp Vitamin E Oil
- Add rose pedals
- Soap molds

Directions:

1. Melt Aloe Vera base soap in the crock-pot or double boiler.
2. When the Aloe Vera completely melt, add oils.
3. pour the mixture in soap molds the add rose pedal
4. on top
5. Once the soap bars are hardened, you can pop them out.

Homemade Shea Butter conditioner

Ingredients:

- ¼ cup Shea Butter or Mango butter
- 3 tsp jojoba
- 2 tsp aloe Vera juice
- 5 drops Rosemary
- 5 drops Lavender
- 2tsp Vitamin E

Directions:

1. Use a double boiler, add your Shea butter and jojoba oil in a bowl, and stir until it melts.
2. Then get it off the double boiler, let it sit.
3. When it cools down, whip the mixture up with a hand mixer. Then add aloe juice, essential oil, and Vitamin E and blend it until it becomes creamy.
4. Pour it in a container.

Chamomile leaves in conditioner

Ingredients:

- 2.5-ounce distilled water
- 4 teaspoon Chamomile Hydrosol
- 4.5g Panthenol
- ½ cup rice starch
- 6.2g Vegetable Glycerin
- 0.128oz Xanthan Gum
- 0.3g arrowroot powder
- 10 drops chamomile essential oil
- 10 drops rosemary essential oil

Directions:

1. You mix vegetable, glycerin, and Xanthan gum together in a container.
2. Then add water, rice starch, panthenol, and arrowroot powder until to the mixture.
3. 10 drops chamomile oil, and 10 drops rosemary essential.
4. Pour it into the spray bottle.
5. It will keep your hair hydrated and moist.

Cocoa Butter Conditioner

Ingredients:

- 2 tbs. of cocoa butter or Mango Butter
- 1 tbs. of coconut oil or Avocado oil
- 1tsp honey
- 1tbs wheatgerm oil or Vitamin E

Directions:

1. Use a double-boiler and add butter, honey, and oil in it.
2. When the mixture has melted, get the double boiler off and let it sit.
3. When it cools down, then whip the mixture up with a hand mixer for 5 minutes.
4. Pour it into a container.
5. Add 5 drops of essential oil (optional).

Turmeric shampoo bar

Ingredients:

- 1 cup Glycerin soap base (Melt and you soap base)
- 1tsp olive oil
- 1tsp honey
- 5-10 drops essential oil (Option)

Second Part:

- ½ cup Glycerin soap base
- ½ cup kokum butter
- 1tsp jojoba oil
- 1tsp honey
- 1tsp turmeric
- 5-10 drops essential oil (Option)

Directions:

1. Put the crockpot, add soap base, and oil; stir it until it melts.
2. Add lemon juices, honey, add vitamin E, keep stirring it well, then pour in your soap mold. Let it sit.

Second Part:

1. Add soap base, honey, oils turmeric, then you pour it on top of another mixture.
2. Let it sit overnight or until harden, then pop them out.

Glycerin shampoo bar

Ingredients:

- 1 cup Glycerin soap base
- 1 tsp avocado oil
- 1 tsp jojoba oil
- 1tsp yucca root powder
- 10 drops lavender essential oil
- 10 drops patchouli essential oil

Directions:

1. Put the crock-pot, add soap base, and oil. Keep stirring it until it melts.
2. Add oils and mix it until the yucca powder becomes solid.
3. Add essential oil and keep stirring it.
4. Pour it in the mold and allow it to harden and pop them out.

Goat milk Shampoo Bar

Ingredients:

- 1 pound goat milk soap base
- 4 tsp honey
- 1 tsp sweet almond
- 5 drops lavender essential oil

Directions:

1. Goat milk soap base (cut small cubes) melt in crock-pot on low then pour the honey in keep stirring it. Add the argan oil and sweet almond oil. Then add vitamin E.
2. Then pour the mixture into the soap molds.
3. When they are completely hardened. You can pop them out and ready to use.

Goat milk Activated Charcoal Shampoo Bar

Ingredients:

- 1 pound goat milk soap base
- 2 tsp activated charcoal-based
- 1tsp baking soda
- 5 drops lemon essential oil

Directions:

1. Goat milk soap base (cut small cubes) melt in crock-pot on low then pour the Activated Charcoal in keep stirring it.
2. Add the baking soda and lemon oil.
3. Then pour the mixture into the soap molds. When they are completely hardened.
4. You can pop them out and ready to use.

Gingerbread Shampoo bar

Ingredients:

- 1 cup Shea butter soap base
- 2tsp jojoba oil
- 1tsp ground ginger
- 1tsp cinnamon
- 5 drops ginger and cinnamon essential oil
- 1 tsp vanilla extract

Directions:

1. Put the crock-pot, add soap base, and oil; stir it until it melts. (Melt in the microwave using 60 seconds, use a good container)
2. Add oils and mix it with ginger and cinnamon.
3. Add vanilla and keep stirring it.
4. Pour it in the mold and allow it to harden and pop them out.

Shea Butter shampoo bar

Ingredients:

- 1 cup Shea butter soap base
- 1 tsp sunflower oil
- 1 tsp jojoba oil
- 1tsp yucca root powder
- 10 drops bergamot oil
- 10 drops ylang-ylang essential oil

Directions:

1. Put the crock-pot, add soap base, and oil. Keep stirring until it melts.
2. Add oils and mix it. Keep stirring until the yucca powder mix well.
3. Add essential oil, keep stirring it.
4. Pour it in the mold and allow it to harden and pop them out.

Oatmeal shampoo bar

Ingredients:

- 1 cup Oatmeal soap base
- 1 tsp argan oil
- 1 tsp jojoba oil
- 1tsp yucca root powder
- 10 drops chamomile essential oil

Directions:

5. Put the crock-pot, add soap base, and oil; stir it until it melts.
6. Add oils and mix it until it melts.
7. Add essential oil, keep stirring it.
8. Pour it in the mold and allow it to harden and pop them out.

Coffee shampoo bars

Ingredients:

- 2cup Goat milk soap base
- 1 tsp argan oil
- 1 tsp jojoba oil
- 1tsp coffee grounds
- 1tsp coffee seed oil
- 0.4 oz espresso fragrance oil

Directions:

1. Put the crock-pot, add soap base, and oil. Keep stirring until it melts.
2. Add oils and keep mixing it.
3. Add essential oil and add the coffee grounds. Keep stirring the mixture.
4. Pour it in the mold and allow it to harden and pop them out.

Sunflower hair scalp oil

Ingredients:

- 2.0 oz Sunflower Seed Oil
- oz Organic Argan Oil
- 2 tbsp Sweet Almond Oil
- 1 tbsp Castor Oil

Directions:

1. Pour it into a bottle and shake well.
2. Massage oil onto the scalp for 2-3 minutes.
3. Continue to use the oil twice a week, depending on the dryness of your hair and scalp.

Fenugreek and Moringa hair Growth oil

Directions:

1. Get a glass container, put ¼ cup argan or grape seed oil in it.
2. Then add 1tsp fenugreek and 1tsp. Moringa with the oils.
3. Put it in a pot to make a double-boiler and put the glass container with ingredients in the water for 5 minutes.
4. Take it off stove, let it cool down so you can strain it.
5. Add 7 drops of rosemary and 7 drops of lavender oil. You can now apply it onto your scalp.

Henna & Amla Powder Hair growth oil

Ingredients:

- 1tsp henna-herbal-hair-color age 12 up or fenugreek oil
- 1tsp Amla Powder
- ½ cup grapeseed or olive oil

Directions:

1. Put it in a glass bottle, let it stay until the next day.
2. Add 7 drops of rosemary essential, and 7 drops of peppermint.
3. You can put it in your hair for a few hours, then use shampoo, or you can let it be in your hair for a few days. It just depends on the condition of your scalp.

Hair Growth blend oil

Ingredients:

- 2 drops thyme essential oil
- 5 drops lavender essential oil
- 5 drops rosemary essential oil
- 2 tbsp grape-seed oil

Directions:

1. Massage the blend into the scalp and let it rest for 20 minutes.
2. Shampoo it out.

Flax seed oil

Ingredients:

- 1 cup flax seed
- 1 cup olive oil

Directions:

1. Get 1 cup flax seeds and blend it.

2. Do a double boil, put your 1 cup of oil in the pot, add your flax seeds. Keep stirring until it changes color, and then strain it.

3 Put it in a container.

4. It is ready to used (It can be used as hot oil, too. Apply on your scalp).

Fenugreek Seed Hair Growth Oil

Ingredients:

- 2 teaspoon Fenugreek seed
- 1tsp grape-seed oil
- 1tsp black castor oil or avocado oil

Directions:

1. Put it in container with all your ingredients for overnight.
2. Strain it the next day.
3. Ready to use, you can now apply it onto your scalp.

Scalp Essential Oils

Ingredients:

- Peppermint oil improves circulation
- lavender oil
- lemon oil promotes healthy hair growth.
- tea tree oil helps improve dandruff
- Rosemary oil reduces hair loss, strengthens hair, and eliminates dandruff and unclogs block hair follicles.
- grapefruit oil
- Sunflower seeds (faster hair growth and help with vitamin E)

Directions:

1. You have to rub essential oils on your hair; it will help with your hair growth.
2. You have to put 5 to 10 drops of oil on your fingertips and massage it on your scalp.
3. Put it in your buttercream or hair grease. You can add this to your shampoo and conditioners.
4. Rosemary and jojoba oil or olive oil are great for hair.

Chamomile Scalp spray

Ingredient:

- 1 tea chamomile
- 1 cup water

Directions:

1. Heat the water and put the tea bag inside.
2. Let it cool down.
3. Put it in your spray bottle.
4. Spray your hair.

Aloe Vera Hair spray

Ingredients:

- 1 cup aloe vera
- 2tsp cloves
- 10 oz distilled water
- 5 drop lavender

Directions:

1. Get a pot and put 10 oz distilled water in it, then pour the cloves (heat on low) for 20mins.
2. Strain it and let it cool down.
3. Add the aloe vera with cloves.
4. Stir the mixture and then add essential oils.
5. Pour it in a spray bottle.

Scalp Spray

Ingredients:

- ¼ cup fresh thyme
- 1 tablespoon of honey
- 1/2 cup raw apple cider vinegar

Directions:

1. Add the thyme leaves in a glass jar.
2. Pour the apple cider vinegar over the leaves. Add the lid.
3. Let the thyme leaves sit for 2-3 days.
4. After three days, strain the leaves and pour into a cup. Spray your scalp as needed.
5. It will get rid of dandruff. Help with hair growth. Use it daily if needed.

Rose Water Treatment Hair Spray For Damaged Hair

Ingredients:

- 1 cup of rose water
- Few drops of jojoba oil
- 1 capsule of vitamin E

Directions:

1. Mix ingredients and apply to wet hair and scalp. Massage for at least 10 min, then you can shampoo and style your hair.

Rosemary and lavender scalp spray

Ingredients:

- 1 cup of distilled water
- 10 drops of rosemary
- 10 drops of lavender
- 1 capsule of vitamin E

Directions:

1. When you get done mix all the ingredient put it in your spray.
2. Message on your scalp then style your hair.

Kids oil

Ingredients:

- 1 cup of grapeseed oil
- 1 tsp baking soda
- 10 drops lavender

Directions:

1. Get a glass bottle (dark), add the oils, then shake it up.

Important: When doing kids' hair, you have to use oil on the hair, not the scalp, if your child's hair is sensitive. Then you seal with one of the butters on the end of the hair. Using water on the child's scalp can also help with growth, not the much 1 or 2 times a week. It just depends on the child's scalp because you don't want it to be too dry. Putting the child in style, just leaving it alone will help with growth. Don't do it all the time; it will cause breakage.

Kids oil

Ingredients:

- ½ olive oil or coconut oil
- 1 tsp avocado
- tsp honey
- 10 drop lavender oil
- 10 drop rosemary oil

Directions:

1. Get a glass or bottle (dark), add the oils and then shake it up. It helps with hair growth.

Onion Juice for hair growth

When using onion juice, it contains sulfur that boosts your collagen production in the tissues. It helps in re-growth of your hair. It does have a strong smell, so leave it on for an hour, then rinse, or you can leave it on longer. It depends on your scalp. Every 4-6 hours after every 4 days.

How to use Onion Juice for your hair?

First, cut a piece of onion and squeeze all the juice out of the onion. Then, you grate it and apply it on a little portion of the scalp until you do the whole head. You leave it on for 10-15 minutes. Just let everything work itself, then rinse it and apply mild shampoo and rinse all done. You will feel refresh.

Coconut Milk Hair Spray (hair grow)

Ingredients:

- You can buy the can or fresh coconut.
- ½ cup coconut milk
- ½ lemon juice
- 4 drops of essential oil
- 6 drops lavender oil

Directions:

1. Mix it thoroughly and apply it to your scalp.
2. Leave it for 4-5 hours (put a hair cap on your head), then rinse it off.

Ayurvedic Herbs - Alma Shikakai Reetha- For Long And Strong Hair

Indian gooseberry (amla) is well-recognized as the powerhouse of vitamin C and antioxidants. Thus, it helps in the production of collagen and also fights off free radicals promoting hair growth and even improving the pigmentation of your hair. You can simply mix 2 teaspoons each of amla powder and lime juice and rub this on your scalp. After some time, rinse with warm water. This will help your hair grow. There is, however, another herbal remedy using amla which can promote faster hair growth by making your hair long, strong, and shiny. For this, you'll have to make a shampoo at home using amla, shikakai, and reetha.

To make amla, shikakai, and reetha shampoo, you will need:

- Amla or Indian gooseberry (Emblica Officinalis) – 100 gm
- Shikakai (Fruit of Acacia concinna shrub) – 100 gm
- Reetha or soapnut (Sapindus Mukorossi) – 100 gm
- Water – 2 liters

Directions:

1. Soak all the three herbs- amla, shikakai, and reetha – in water overnight.
2. In the morning, boil the mixture till the time water reduces to half.
3. Let it cool.
4. Once the mixture cools, with the help of hands, mash the boiled herbs to a pulp in the water itself.
5. Now strain and collect the homemade shampoo in another utensil.
6. Wash your hair with this shampoo.
7. Do not try to rub the herbal liquid as you do when using regular shampoos. This will entangle your hair leading to breakage as your hair goes rough as soon as it comes in contact with this herbal shampoo.

Rose scalp Oils

Ingredients:

- Dry roses
- ½ cup sunflower oil

Directions:

1. Put roses in a glass container with the oil, then get a pot and fill it with water.
2. Place the glass container inside 45 mins and let it cool.
3. Repeat the process.
4. Strain the roses and put it in a glass container.

Herbal scalp oil

Ingredients:

- 1 cup curry leave
- 1 cup tulsi
- tsp fenugreek seeds
- 1 cup mustard oil
- 1 cup neem oil
- 1 cup badam oil
- 1 cup sunflowers oil

Directions:

1. Put the curry leaves, tulsi, fenugreek seeds in a glass bowl with the oils then get a pot full it with water a place the glass container inside 45 mins.
2. Strain it let it cool down.
3. Put it in a container.

Onion scalp oil

Ingredients:

- 2 onions
- 1cup sunflower oil

Directions:

1. Put the Onion in a glass container with oil.
2. Then get a pot and fill it with water and place the glass container inside 45 mins.
3. Strain the onion and put it in a glass container.
4. Then apply on scalp.

Ginger scalp oil

Ingredients:

- ½ cup ginger
- 1 cup avocado oil
- add few cloves(optional)

Directions:

1. Put the ginger in a glass container with oil.
2. Now get a pot, fill it with water, and place the glass container inside refrigerator for 1 hour.
3. Strain the ginger and put it in a glass container.

Substitute Oil and Butters

Low Porosity oil

Argan oil

Grape seed oil

Jojoba oil

Rose hip oil

Safflower oil

Baobab oil

Apricot oil

Avocado oil

Camela seed oil

Pomegranate oil

Sweet almond oil

High Porosity oil

Coconut oil

Hemp seed oil

Castor oil

Olive oil

Moringa oil

Jojoba oil

Mustard oil

Low Porosity Butter	High Porosity Butter
Monoi Butter	Ucuubba Butter
Avocado Butter	Shea Butter
Cocoa Butter	Kokum Butter
Cupuacu Butter	Mango Butter
Tucuman Butter	
Babassu Butter	
Muru Butter	

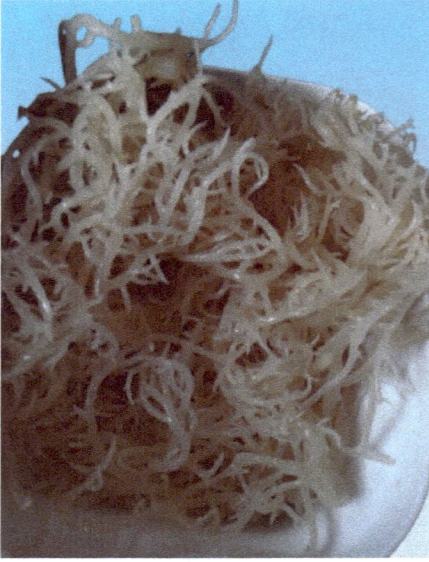

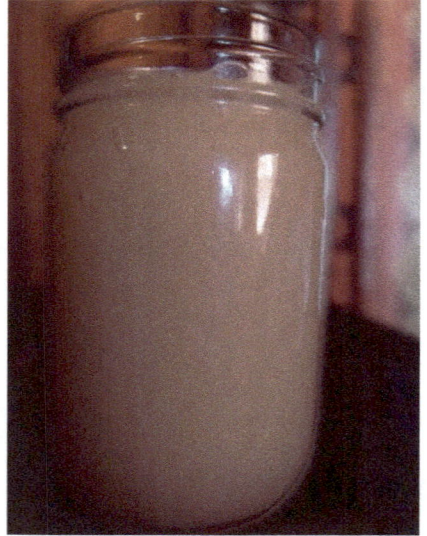

Sea Moss

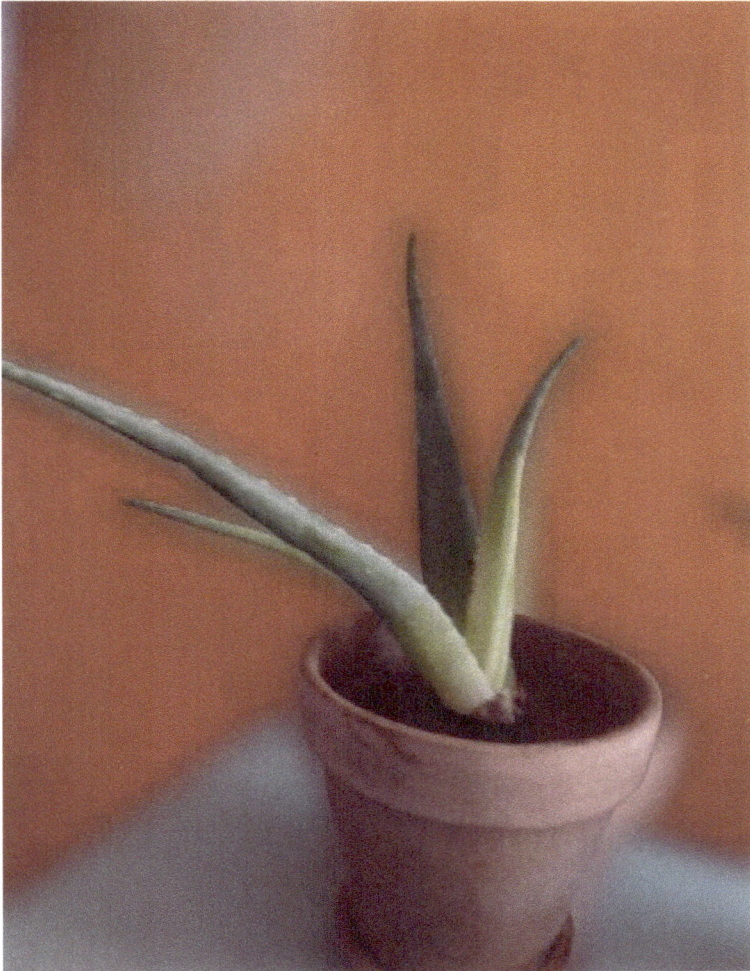

Aloe Vera Plant

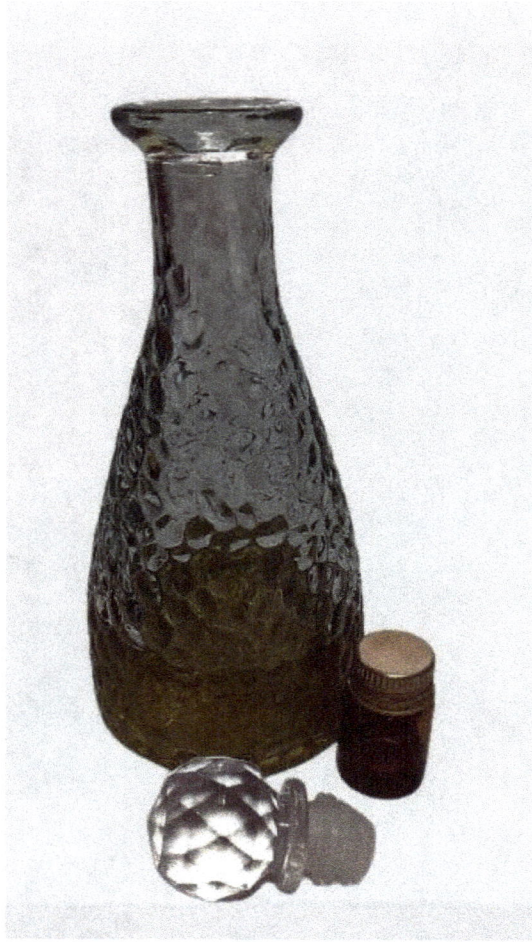

Hair Oil

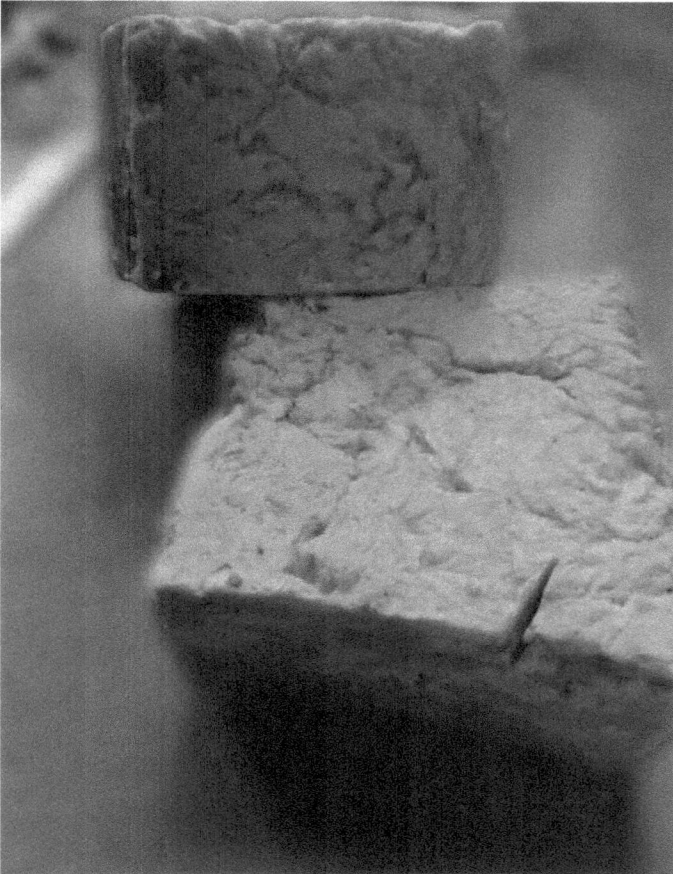

Pumpkin Spice Shampoo Bar

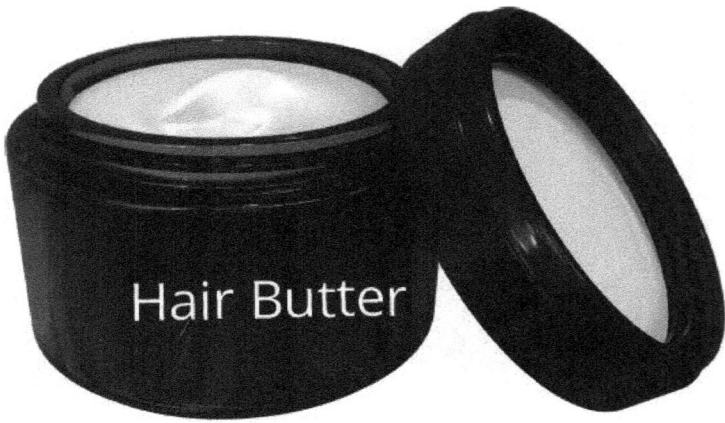